Linda V. Yelton

The Yamas and Niyamas

A yogic path to your higher self and manifestation

Balboa Press books may be ordered through booksellers or by contacting:

Balboa Press
A Division of Hay House
1663 Liberty Drive
Bloomington, IN 47403
www.balboapress.com
844-682-1282

ISBN: 978-1-9822-6706-3 (sc)
978-1-9822-6707-0 (e)

Library of Congress Control Number: 2021907305

Print information available on the last page.

Balboa Press rev. date: 06/08/2021

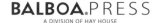

BALBOA.PRESS
A DIVISION OF HAY HOUSE

The Yamas and Niyamas

A yogic path to your
higher self and manifestation

Table of Contents

Introduction

I recall winning at swimming. I would dive into the pool, reach out and pull the other side to me.

When I was between 10 and 17, I swam for the local swimming pool's team, the North Springfield Dolphins. I was a very fast swimmer. Nevertheless, sometimes I would allow a teammate to beat me during time-trials just because they needed it more than I did, or rather, because I wanted to feel their joy. During a time-trial race, I'd be swimming in the lane next to my teammate, keeping pace but easily able to pull ahead. We'd swim beside each other evenly, but at the last tenth of a second, I'd pull back a bit and let them touch the wall first. I'd still come in second, fast enough to be selected to compete in the upcoming swimming meet where I would place within the first three in every event.

During the swimming meets, when it came to the relays, I knew I was swimming for the rest of the team, so I never let anyone beat me. Because of that, the coaches always put me at anchor no matter where I'd placed in time trials and no matter what the relay: medley relay, put Linda at anchor; freestyle relay, put Linda at anchor; 200 meters, 100 meters put Linda at anchor. The coaches knew that I would win no matter what. Invariably, the three swimmers who preceded me on my relay team would fall behind their opposing swimmer. At times, they would touch the wall after the opposition was halfway down the pool. Miraculously, I always beat them and won for the team.

I remember the feeling of diving into the water and seeming to reach to the other side of the pool and pull it to me. I did it in perfect faith, without any doubt about the outcome. I was, at those times, completely joined with my higher self, with infinite source energy. I came to the relay with the mind of a child, who accepts the given without any doubt. Indeed, I came to the swim team as a child whose primary value was the experience of joy in everyone because, intuitively, I knew that we are all one.

As time passed, I became aware of limitations that were put on me and others by the opinions, expectations and pressures of society. I started to doubt myself. I started to envy other people. I started to worry about what others thought of me. And I started to judge others as well. Life became a struggle that I accepted because I thought that life is supposed to be a struggle. I thought that you had to strive and suffer to achieve what you want in life. But nothing could be further from the truth. The truth is that infinite source energy is ready, at all times, to deliver to you that which you most desire, indeed, that which resonates with your higher self. And that which resonates with your higher self *is* the thing you most desire. It is that thing that makes your heart sing when you think about it and makes you dance with joy when you realize it.

But as life flows through time, we lose our ability to see infinite source and feel as if we are our higher self. Just as a ripple on water distorts the surface such that you cannot see through to the bottom of the water, so too do limiting thoughts, opinions, expectations, and doubt create ripples on the surface of the mind to distort your ability to see through to infinite source.

Yoga provides a way to smooth the surface of our mind, beginning with the Yoga principles called the Yamas and practices called the Niyamas.

Chapter 1

Yoga is the Sanskrit root of the English word yoke. A yoke is a type of harness that joins two animals together to leverage their strength. It is typically made of a wooden beam with loops that go around the animals' heads. It is normally used between a pair of oxen or other animals to enable them to pull together on a load when working in pairs, as oxen usually do.

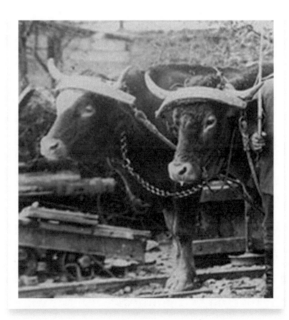

The word Yoga literally means to yoke together with infinite source. Yoga is a practice that joins you to infinite source. It is far more than group fitness or a good stretch. In fact, when practiced as intended, Yoga can help you enter the field of your dreams. Yoga lets you connect easily with the things, people and events that you desire. Yoga is the practice that leads that field and that connection. But most people do not know this about Yoga. They think of Yoga as group exercise or a good stretch. At the end of a Yoga class, when they are asked to rest for a few minutes in corpse pose, they lie there with their minds racing, unable to calm the thoughts that pass through.

Most modern Western Yoga classes typically teach only the third limb of the path, posture or "asana" which is called "Yoga" in our culture. Some classes teach the fourth limb: pranayama or breath control.

I remember once a few years ago, at the end of the Yoga class that I taught in Northern Virginia, a young woman came up to me and asked, "How can I calm my mind? Each time I try to meditate, I can't get the mind chatter to stop. I follow my breath and do what I'm supposed to do, but the mind chatter just continues."

I said, "Funny you are asking me this now because I have been thinking about meditation and the way that it is taught in Yoga classes."

At that time, I'd been practicing Transcendental Meditation since I was 19—a long time ago—when the Maharishi Mahesh Yogi brought the practice to the U.S. for the first time. Yet, I still struggled. My solution was to use a mantra.

A mantra is a sacred, a numinous sound, a syllable, word or group of words that some believe to have spiritual powers.

The earliest mantras are composed in Vedic Sanskrit and have been used for thousands of years. In sophisticated forms, mantras are melodic phrases with spiritual interpretations such as a human longing for truth, reality, light, immortality, peace, love, knowledge, and action. Some mantras without literal meaning are musically uplifting and spiritually meaningful. At its simplest, the word Om (Aum) may serve as a mantra. In Yoga, Om is taught to be the first sound which was originated on earth. Om sound is said to create a reverberation in the body which helps the body and mind to be calm.

So this is what I answered to young woman: "When you are trying to meditate and the mind chatter takes over, replace it with the sound 'Om'. Use the sound 'Om' to replace any monkey mind chatter as it comes about. Say it in your mind, or you can even say it out loud at first if you want. When you start to hear your mind going over your grocery list, or rehearsing what you are going to tell someone, just replace the sound of that chatter with the sound of Om, repeating Om over and over exchanging it for the intruding chatter."

"Thanks," she said, and walked away.

But what I told her to do is not meditation. It is a technique of the practice of "Transcendental Meditation" to replace the chatter with the sound of your mantra—your individual mantra.

This technique isn't the meditation itself. It is preparatory to meditation and will eventually bring your mind to a state where it is empty, for brief moments at first, and then meditation begins. From your empty mind, you access the infinite—you yoke to the infinite source—and this is meditation. Accessing the infinite source of creation in meditation is the natural outcome of Yoga.

> *Yet, it can be nearly impossible to empty your mind and*
> *free it from mind chatter when you are feeling guilt, shame,*
> *victimhood, revenge or any other fear-based emotion.*

Practicing the Yamas and Niyamas frees your mind of such chatter. It is the intention of this book to explain why and how to practice to achieve a clear mind that allows you to yoke to the infinite.

Learning to meditate according to Patanjali's Yoga Sutra is a deep practice, with several stages, including an eight-limbed path that forms the structural framework for the Yoga practice. The eight limbs are progressive stages preparing for meditation and Samadhi. The eight limbs begin with the Yamas and the Niyamas.

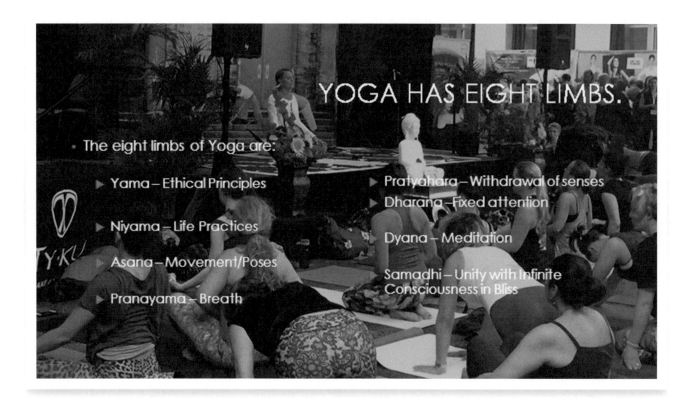

YOGA HAS EIGHT LIMBS.

The eight limbs of Yoga are:

▶ Yama – Ethical Principles

▶ Niyama – Life Practices

▶ Asana – Movement/Poses

▶ Pranayama – Breath

▶ Pratyahara – Withdrawal of senses

▶ Dharana – Fixed attention

Dyana – Meditation

Samadhi – Unity with Infinite Consciousness in Bliss

They progress through Asana (poses), Pranayama or breath control. The next four limbs are Pratyahara, the withdrawal of senses, Dharana, fixed attention, Dyana, meditation and Samadhi, union with the infinite source of energy.

Pratyahara, the fifth limb of the path, means withdrawal of awareness from the external world of outside stimuli, while directing our attention internally. This practice allows us to step back and take a look at ourselves objectively observing our habits and encouraging our inner growth. Pratyahara prepares for the next limb, Dharana.

Dharana teaches us how to slow down the thinking process by concentrating on a single mental object, a specific energetic center in the body, an image of a deity, or the silent repetition of a sound, such as the mantra practice that I described to the young woman

(". . .use the sound Om to replace any monkey mind chatter as it comes about") is a practice of Dharana.

Dhyana, the next limb is meditation. Where Dharana is one-pointed attention, dhyana is ultimately a state of being keenly aware without focus. At this stage, the mind has been quieted, and in the stillness it produces few or no thoughts at all.

The final limb is Samadhi. At this stage, the yogi or yogini merges with his or her point of focus and transcends the self altogether. This is where you "yoke" to infinite source energy. This is where you meet your higher self and access the fifth dimension where all being exists unchanged until it is syntropically drawn to existence in our three dimensions, limited by the fourth dimension of time.

It is living according to the teachings of the Yamas and Niyamas that allows us to develop a Yoga practice leading to a calm mind.

Let's a deep look at the Yamas and Niyamas. We will examine each of these ethical principles and how each of the practices support them. In doing so, we will discover how to employ the Yamas and Niyamas in our daily life to calm our minds and reach the state of surrender to our higher self where the fifth dimensional field of all possibilities opens before us.

First, though, let me introduce myself as more than a childhood-competitive swimmer and adult Yoga teacher. I was born in Chicago, but I was raised the Washington, DC suburbs. I earned a BA in Psychology from George Mason University. I've had a long career conducting and analyzing consumer and industry research for such organizations as McDonald's restaurant chain, George Soros's Open Society Institute, and major US industry associations. Known as a "China Expert" from 2000 through 2010, the results of my primary research projects have been used to make policy decisions by the governments of the US, Sweden, and the EU.

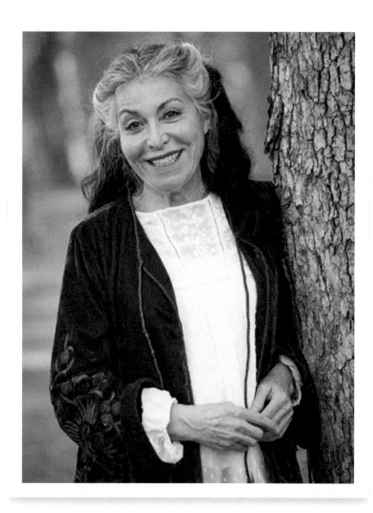

This career path was not satisfying to me. Indeed, it was frustrating as it was all superficial.

I've been on a spiritual quest since early childhood. My parents raised me to give me exposure to many of mankind's religions and sacred traditions, while opening my mind to fearless curiosity. Unfortunately, mid-century America did not make it easy to find spiritual information that went beyond Judeo-Christian dogma. In fact, it seemed as if all other knowledge was called occult or even witchcraft, making it all-the-more attractive to me!

As a teenage hippie, I started to follow the same path as Richard Alpert whom you may know today as Ram Dass. Alpert was an associate of Timothy Leary, an early researcher into psychedelics. "Turn on, Tune in, Drop out" was Leary's mantra and I was "all in." I learned from following the teachings of Ram Dass and Timothy Leary to open the portal to the "all there is," revealing to me that "all" is energy, I am one with energy and can fuse with infinite energy, or not, as I will. You see, I discovered that my immediate environment is completely under my own control. Yet, I was chagrined to realize that most people believe that they are controlled by the rules of authorities, society, even the rules of existence itself, unaware that all those rules are games, pure and simple. I longed to enlighten those around me, but I didn't know how.

I turned to Transcendental Meditation as taught by the Beatles' guru, the Maharishi Mahesh Yogi. Despite his title Yogi, I did not realize that the meditative practice he taught is the final limb of Yoga, best achieved through mastery of the preceding seven limbs of Yoga. Thus, even with my own personal mantra, achieving the true meditative state (samadhi) was a struggle.

At the same time, I earned a degree in Jungian Psychology from George Mason University and went on to graduate school under the same Jungian teacher. I learned archetypes, synchronicity, the collective unconscious, and even started casting I Ching coins to predict the future for other students. I studied the Tao Te Ching, The Tibetan Book of the Dead, The Bhagavad Gita, Philosophia Hermetica, the Bible, and any other ancient texts I could get my hands on. I studied the work of Madame Blavatsky, Aleister Crowley, Manley Hall, Ophiel, Starhawk, Anton LaVey and more.

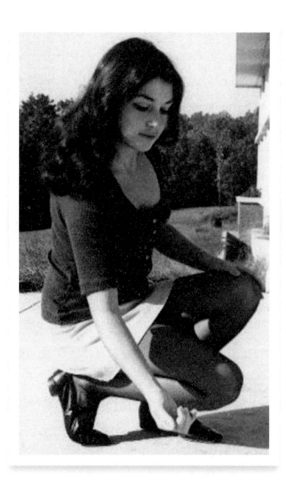

And then, in mid-life, someone taught me human energetics and how to clear my chakra. Bringing chakra clearing into my meditative practice opened the astral field to me and I was able to perceive guidance from the infinite. Yet again, I didn't realize this was Yoga!

Fast forward through life, I finally came to the physical practice of Yoga known as Asana, the second limb. I was lucky enough to land in a studio whose owner taught Yoga as both a physical and spiritual practice. It seemed each asana class I took opened me to myself, layer by layer, and I realized Yoga was a path to what I had been seeking all my life. So I took Yoga teacher training, learned the eight limbs, and the puzzle pieces fell into place. Yoga ties it all together and provides a path to enlightenment by following the eight limbs, mastering them one at a time in sequence.

In 2010, I became a certified, Registered Yoga Teacher.

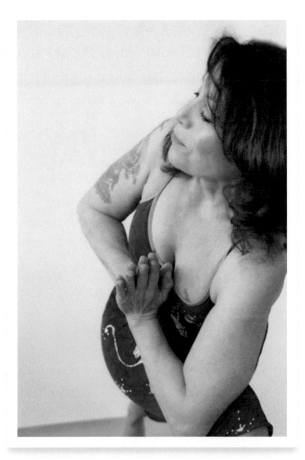

Only now do I feel competent to try to enlighten people to their own power. The way to do so, I believe, is to teach the ancient wisdom of the Yoga that says if you want to discover your higher self and become one with the source of all there is, then live according to the tenets of the Yamas and the Niyamas.

I wrote this book as an introduction to the principles and practices that lead the Yogi or Yogini to experience union with infinite source and meet their higher self. The Yamas and Niyamas provide a road map to "union with infinite source" this practice leads to the the field of "all there is". We draw our manifestations from that field.

Little did I know many years ago, when I won those swimming relays, that I did so from the infinite field. My child's mind was uncluttered so I could access my higher self and draw to my physical self the energy of winning. It has taken me a lifetime to understand where the energy came from and how to draw upon it. Now, I want to teach you to do the same.

Chapter 2

The universe is of the nature of a thought or sensation in a universal Mind. To put the conclusion crudely – the stuff of the world is mind-stuff. As is often the way with crude statements, I shall have to explain that by "mind" I do not exactly mean mind and by "stuff" I do not at all mean stuff. Still that is about as near as we can get to the idea in a simple phrase. Sir Arthur Eddington, British Astronomer.

"Yogas citta vrtti nerodha." Translated: Yoga is the calming of the fluctuations of the mind stuff. Second Yoga Sutra of Patanjali

Yoga leads us to perceive the universal mind—the source of infinite possibilities that exist, at once, waiting to manifest into our three-dimensional world, over time, upon our observation. How does this work?

Let's begin to look at the concept of fifth-dimension, which in physics, is the realm of all possibilities. We may start with the story of "Schroedinger's Cat."

Erwin Schroedinger, was an Austrian-Irish, Nobel Prize winning physicist who developed and furthered the field quantum theory. He famously proposed a thought experiment to disprove the idea that observation is the cause of manifestation. In quantum physics terms, manifestation is worded as "a superposition collapsing into one state."

In Schroedinger's thought experiment, a cat is placed in a box with a tiny bit of radioactive substance. When the radioactive substance decays, it triggers a Geiger counter, which releases a poison that kills the cat. But since there is no conscious observer present (everything is in a sealed box), the cat remains both dead and alive at the same time—in a superposition—until the box is opened and observed. Once observed, the cat becomes either dead or alive.

SCHRÖDINGER'S CAT

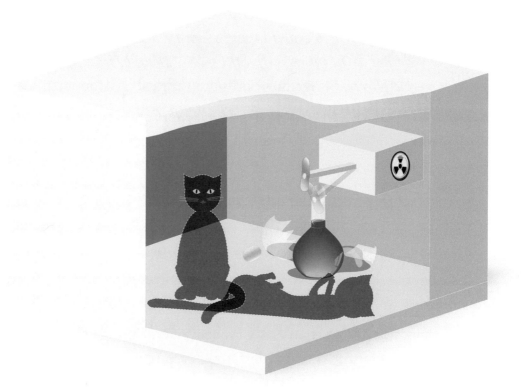

Schroedinger proposed that the existence of a cat that is both dead and alive at the same time is absurd and does not happen in the "real" world. He believed that this thought experiment proved that the outcome of events is not driven by observation. However, over time, this thought experiment has been used to demonstrate just the opposite. As long as the box is closed, we cannot know if the cat is dead or alive. It could be either dead or alive, thus remains in a superposition—both states at once—until it is observed.

The cat's superposition exists in the fifth dimension. The fifth dimension is the dimension in which everything is in a static superposition until it is observed. Let me explain.

We are taught that we live in a three-dimensional universe bound by time. These dimensions are, first, a line, which extended becomes the second, dimension—a plane, when extended becomes the third dimension—a cube, a sphere or some other solid shape. Moving the solid through space, we experience time, considered the fourth dimension.

Our experience of these dimensions goes something like this: you and I agree to meet in the mezzanine lobby of the building at the corner of Fifth and Elm at 3 PM Tuesday. Thus, we have set a space and time to meet. Both of us have to move through three dimensions at a particular time to arrive in a certain space.

Or we may be sitting at the dinner table when you might say to me, "pass the potatoes." I hand over the solid bowl of potatoes to your place over the course of a few seconds of time.

Modern day physics tells us that the universe has a fifth dimension where everything is static, not moving or changing over time, but remaining in one state. It is said to be invisible because it is a micro-dimension, too small for us to perceive and it is thought to be curled into itself in a spiral. Unlike our familiar three dimensions, bound by time, where entropy, i.e decay, is always increasing, in the fifth dimension, entropy doesn't exist. In the fifth dimension, everything, every possibility, exists without change until it is perceived and manifested into our three-dimensional reality in a moment in time.

This idea is derived from quantum theory, which goes further to propose the idea that the fifth dimension is always in a state of "quantum superposition." That is, quantum particles, the building blocks of solids, may be in more than one state of being at the same time and collapse down to a single state upon interaction with other particles. Many physicists believe that quantum particles only collapse to a single state when viewed by a conscious observer, thus melding quantum theory with the teachings of ancient philosophies, such as Yoga.

Considering the fifth dimension, its lack of entropy plus its constant state of superposition, we can look at the fifth dimension as a field of possibilities that come to fruition only upon observation. Observation happens at each moment in time. In the fifth dimension, each possibility exists unchanged until it is observed and manifested in our three-dimensional world over tme. Thus, as you are pushing through the leading edge of time, moment by moment, your observation causes each possibility to unfold in three dimensions.

But because most of us have minds that are cluttered by random thoughts, we never realize that our observation is manifesting our world. The chattering nature of our thoughts prevents us from seeing into the fifth dimension. Our minds are filled with ponderings that prattle on about our "to-do list," our grievances, our fears. These haphazard thoughts are like the ripples on the surface of water that prevent us from seeing through it. When we practice Yoga, we calm these ripples and create a clear surface where we can see all possible outcomes in the superposition of the fifth dimension as if they are in "front" of us.

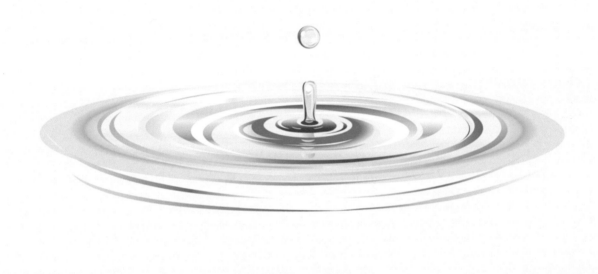

Practicing Yoga means more than just posing. When practiced in our daily life, the Yamas and Niyamas help us to calm the mind and lead us to a state of surrender to our higher self where the fifth dimension becomes not only perceivable but where our observations manifest our intentions. The Yamas and Niyamas actually guide us along a path that leads to the fifth dimension.

My intention with this book is to provide a foundation from which to build your own spiritual practice and knowledge to bring you into contact with the infinite, the "all there is." It is from that position that all things manifest, including your intentions." Yoga can lead you to that position.

Chapter 3

As my Yoga practice progressed, I have studied with most of the American Masters, including Rodney Yee, Dharma Mittra, Shiva Rhea, and others. Over time, I came to see the physical practice as leading to meditation, and finally gained an understanding of what Yoga is.

Teaching showed me the importance of emphasizing that Yoga is not just physical, but it is a lifestyle that leads to contentment and so much more.

Yoga has eight limbs, as mentioned in the previous chapter. It is not just the physical practice of Asana. Yoga's eight limbs include a set of ethical principles and practices that lead to peace of mind.

As mentioned in a previous chapter, the eight limbs begin with the Yamas and the Niyamas. They progress through Asana (poses), Pranayama or breath control. The next four limbs are Pratyahara, the withdrawal of senses, Dharana, fixed attention, Dyana, meditation and Samadhi, union with the infinite source of energy.

This book will, hopefully, lead you into a much deeper understanding of the Yamas as ethical guidance and the Niyamas as ethical practices. The Yamas and Niyamas are the first two limbs.

Most people in the western world start with Asana and many never learn that Yoga is so much more. If a western Yoga class does introduce the ethical principles, called the Yamas, usually they focus on Ahimsa, saying that if you are a vegetarian, you are practicing Ahimsa.

In an Asana class, we usually end with Savasana or corpse pose, in which we are asked to practice Pratyahara, Dharana and Dyana; we are asked to meditate. And this is where modern Western Yogis have problems. They cannot calm their minds.

Like the ripples on the surface of water that make it impossible to see clearly to the bottom of the body of water, mind chatter makes it impossible to see clearly through to infinite consciousness. When the mind is constantly rehearsing revenge scripts and feeling victimhood, it is impossible to calm.

When those thoughts are eliminated by living ethically, according to the principles and practices of the Yamas and Niyamas, the mind is clear and able to see through to the infinite.

The Yamas and Niyamas were introduced to Yoga by an ancient Yoga master named Patanjali in his **Yoga Sutras** sometime between 5,000 and 2,500 years ago. Legend has it that the **Yoga Sutras** were given to Patanjali from Vishnu, the preserver. Vishnu is one of the three principal Hindu gods, the other two being Bhrama, the creator, and Shiva the destroyer. The **Yoga Sutras** are the set of laws and practices that guide Yoga.

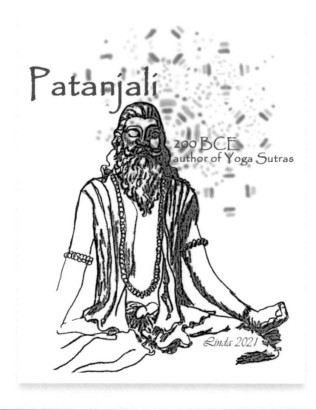

- It is thought his work can be attributed to more than one author.

- The legend of his origin is that Vishnu was lying on the bed of snakes — the serpent Adishésha with a 1,000 heads. When the Rishis approached Him, He gave them Adishésha (the symbol of awareness), who took birth in the world as Maharishi Patanjali.

- Hence Patanjali came to this earth to give this knowledge of Yoga which came to be known as the Yoga Sutras.

The Yoga Sutras provide explanations and guidance in the ethical principles, the Yamas and practices, the Niyamas. They are described as spiritual laws that are eternal. The earliest mention of *Yamas* is found in the Hindu scripture Rigveda, in verse 5.61.2. The word in the Rigveda means a "rein" or "curb," the act of checking or curbing, restraining such as by a charioteer or a driver. Yamas is the Sanskrit word for "restraint," particularly from actions, words, or thoughts that may cause harm The term evolves into a moral restraint and ethical duty.

The Yamas and the Niyamas are often seen as separate, in that the Yamas are how one acts towards others and the Niyamas how one acts toward oneself. But they also work together in that one cannot act one way toward others and another way toward yourself. We all know that it is impossible to love another unless you love yourself. Thus, how can you act with non-violence toward another while you are indulging in self-destructive activities, such as addiction or body mutilation.

> ### *I like to think of the Yamas as the road to achieving union with infinite source energy and the Niyamas the vehicle to get there.*

If that is the case, then the road is paved with Ahimsa. As we go through the Yamas you will see that Ahimsa underpins the other four.

The road leads to the last of the Niyamas, Isvara Pranadana, which is surrender to infinite source. It is in that surrender that one achieves Samadhi. Without surrender, one cannot achieve Samadhi.

It is in surrender to infinite source that one reaches the fifth dimension, the field of syntropy, and finds the power to manifest reality.

So, let's take a deep dive into these principals, starting with Ahimsa, which means non-violence.

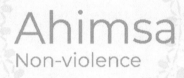

Ahimsa
Non-violence

Chapter 3 Ahimsa— Non Violence

If you practice Asana Yoga, such as Ashtanga or flow, in a studio, you have probably been in a class that was dedicated to Ahimsa. And probably your teacher emphasized veganism. And so you left the class thinking that if you became vegan, you would be practicing Ahimsa. And that's all good. But Ahimsa is so much more. Let's look deeper at Ahimsa.

Book two of Patanjali's *Yoga Sutras*, Chapter 35

♥ ***In the presence of one firmly established in non-violence, all hostilities cease. (translation by Sri Swami Satchidananda)***

♥ **Himsa means pain and A is the opposite. Ahimsa, then, means "not causing pain."**

Ahimsa is the state of non-violence. When the vow of ahimsa is established, all enmity ceases because that person emits harmonious vibrations.

I looked to contemporary Yoga masters to see how they saw Ahimsa. In particular, I chose to look into the teachings of TKV Desikachar and BKV Inyengar because these two are among the most likely to be referenced in modern Yoga teacher training.

Tirumalai Krishnamacharya Venkata Desikachar better known as T. K. V. Desikachar, is the son of the "father of modern Yoga" Tirumalai Krishnamacharya. The style of Yoga that he developed is called Viniyoga, from which the practice of Vinyasa Yoga comes and which is aligned with the *Yoga Sutras* of Patanjali. Desikachar was born in Mysore and moved to Madras (now Chennai) in the early 1960s. Although he had trained as an engineer, he was inspired by his father's teachings, and he studied under his father in the 1960s. He became an international teacher and wrote many books, including **The Heart of Yoga** which is the reference I used to inform this book because it is widely used as a text in modern Western Yoga teacher training.

Bellur Krishnamachar Sundararaja Iyengar better known as B.K.S. Iyengar, is the founder of the style of "Iyengar Yoga" and was considered one of the foremost yoga teachers in the world.

B.K.S. Iyengar was the 11th of 13 children (10 of whom survived) born to Sri Krishnamachar, a school teacher, and Sheshamma. When Iyengar was five years old, his family moved to Bangalore. Four years later, the 9-year-old boy lost his father to appendicitis. Throughout his childhood, he struggled with malaria, tuberculosis, typhoid fever, and general malnutrition.

In 1934, his brother-in-law, the Yogi Sri Tirumalai Krishnamacharya (mentioned above as Desikachar's father) asked the 15-year-old Iyengar to come to Mysore, so as to improve his health through the practice of Yoga asanas. Krishnamacharya had Iyengar and other students give asana demonstrations in the Maharaja's court at Mysore, which had a positive influence on Iyengar. Iyengar considers his association with his brother-in-law a turning point in his life saying that over a two-year period "he (Krishnamacharya) only taught me for about ten or fifteen days, but those few days determined what I have become today!" Krishnamacharya began teaching a series of difficult postures, sometimes telling him to not eat until he mastered a certain posture. These experiences would later inform the way he taught his students. Iyengar reported in interviews that, at age 90, he continued to practice asanas for three hours and pranayamas for an hour daily. Inyengar is the author of many books on yoga practice and philosophy including **Light on Yoga**, which is the reference I used to inform this book because it is widely used as a text in modern Western Yoga teacher training.

- **TKV Desikachar says Ahimsa is more than non-violence, but acting in consideration of the situation. This refers back to the Bhagavad Gita where Arjuna was loath to go to battle, but Krishna reminded him of his dharma.**

Desikachar's reference to the Bhagavad Gita considers dharma. Dharma is our life's purpose within the order of the universe. It is our place within the universe, the roll we play. Karma doesn't really affect that role, but it does affect the expression of that role. Desikachar is here talking about the dilemma one faces when one is asked to live out a dharma that is antithetical to Ahimsa. In this case, it is Arjuna's dharma as a warrior. In the Bhagavad Gita, Krishna tells Arjuna to do the right thing for its own sake without worrying about success or failure. Do your best because that is what destiny demands. Act with grace under pressure.

Iyengar goes a bit deeper in his discussion of Ahimsa.

- **BKS Iyengar says Ahimsa is love that embraces all creation, again taking in the teachings of the Bhagavad Gita. He says that you denounce the violence but not the person doing the violence. He talks about freedom from fear and anger. He says that the Yogi is gentle of mind with others but disciplined with his own mind, referring to discernment of action.**

When he references discernment of action, he asks the yogi to understand the Dharma that is playing out. This is difficult, which is why he asks for gentleness of mind, forgiveness.

I also looked to female Yoga teachers to ensure the feminine perspective was considered. In general, women believe that Ahimsa extends to all of creation, including yourself. The female perspective is that females are mothers and nurturers. To be a good mother is to be good to yourself in that you—your body—brings new life and therefore should be treated with non-violence. We are asked by women to face our inner demons and do the Shadow Work to develop self-love so that we can love those we are called to nurture.

We will go into Shadow work later, but first let's look at the nature of violence.

- ♥ There are only two states of being: Love and Fear

- ♥ Violence is a function of fear.

- ♥ Fear comes from the strong boundaries we impose on ourselves due to materialism or ideology and ego. We violently defend our identity or border.

Of the two states of being, love and fear, fear is driven by the idea that our boundaries are being violated in some way. We defend the boundaries created by our ego, or our space because we identify with these boundaries. We fear if the boundaries are broken or intruded upon we will lose our very identity. Your country, your home, your body are all part of your identity. Without that identity, your very existence ceases to be, doesn't it? So you defend those boundaries with violence often expressed as anger, hatred, jealousy, envy and competition. This violence causes shame, guilt, doubt and even self-loathing. The mind can hardly be calm with that type of stuff going on.

- ♥ Its companions are anger, hatred, jealousy, envy and competition.

- ♥ It causes guilt, shame, doubt, and self loathing, all of which are barriers to our own equanimity.

**The 16ᵗʰ Dalai Lama said, "The true hero
is one who conquers his own anger and hatred."**

So what can we do to conquer those fearful feelings? What can we do to practice ahimsa? We must commit to love over fear.

First we do no harm.

Like doctors who take an oath not to harm, we too can commit to doing no harm. One of the ways Ahimsa is practiced in modern culture is through the Hippocratic oath taken by doctors that says,

- ♥ "As to diseases, make it a habit of two things – to help, or at least do no harm."

  We can develop compassion, learning to act in opposition to fearfulness. The prayer of St. Francis of Assisi is a universal example of developing compassion. (Read the prayer) Lord,

- ♥ Make me an instrument of your peace
- ♥ Where there is hatred. . . let me sow love
- ♥ Where there is injury. . . pardon
- ♥ Where there is discord. . . harmony
- ♥ Where there is doubt. . . faith
- ♥ Where there is despair. . . hope
- ▶ Where there is darkness. . . light
- ▶ Where there is sadness. . . joy

Develop Empathy

- ♥ Empathy is the ability to sense another being's energies, emotions, pain, joy, fear as if it is your own.
- ♥ Empaths often cannot determine their own emotions from those of others.
- ♥ Ahimsa is practiced by feeling another being's fear and acting to reassure that person.

Although we may not all be empaths, we've all felt emotions. When we see another with those emotions, we can remember how we felt. And in that remembering, we develop empathy.

We can feel how another being is feeling by remembering that feeling in our own experience. Have you ever cried during a sad movie? That's empathy.

I asked a social media group of empaths to tell me how they felt empathy. Here are two responses:

> *I can see their thoughts and feelings independent of mine. Others' feelings and thoughts are like a wave beside me that I can reach to and become aware of.*

> *Physically feeling their emotions and imagining myself as I am them. It's like you become them as one and you are experiencing what they are experiencing*

If you cannot feel another's feelings, at least you can then wish them well. You can develop compassion. In Yoga, compassion is a virtue that reaches back to the ancient Vedic texts. In fact, compassion is considered central to Ahimsa. The Dalai Lama once said, "If you want others to be happy, practice compassion. If you want to be happy, practice compassion."

Compassion is the complement to kindness. While kindness wishes the happiness and welfare of another, compassion wishes that others be free from suffering, a wish to be extended without limits to all living beings, including yourself. Indeed, to be compassionate you must be able to experience and fully appreciate your own suffering and to have compassion for yourself.

The Buddha is reported to have said, "It is possible to travel the whole world in search of one who is more worthy of compassion than oneself. No such person can be found."

Forgive

- Forgiveness is for you.
- Holding a grudge binds you to fear and breeds violence.

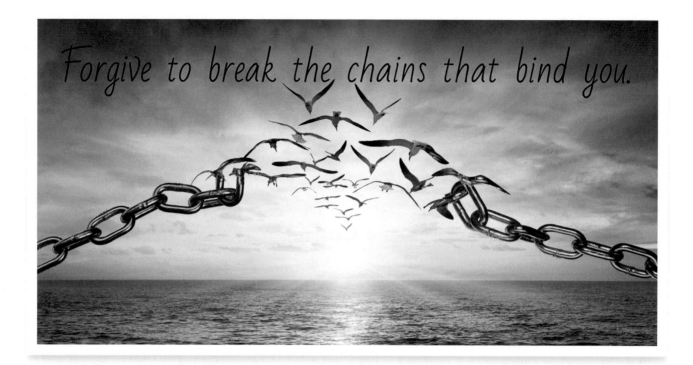

A grudge is the most toxic thing you can hold. No matter how egregious the harm against you, holding on to the hate that crime engendered is worse. It repeats the harm in your experience over and over again. You never get past it, unless you forgive. Forgiving may be the hardest thing you ever do. But it will relieve you of having to relive the event that caused the harm. Forgiveness is for you. It is not for the person who harmed you. It is truly Ahimsa toward yourself.

Follow the Golden Rule.

The Golden Rule seems to be universal. It is seminal and appears in every human religion or spiritual practice under slightly different wording.

- ***Christianity:*** In everything, do to others as you would have them do to you; for this is the law and the prophets. *Jesus, Matthew 7:12*

- ***Buddhism:*** Treat not others in ways that you yourself would find hurtful. *The Buddha, Udana-Varga 5.18*

- ***Hinduism:*** This is the sum of duty: do not do to others what would cause pain if done to you. *Mahabharata 5:1517*

- ***Islam:*** Not one of you truly believes until you wish for others what you wish for yourself. *The Prophet Muhammad, Hadith*

- ***Judaism:*** What is hateful to you, do not do to your neighbour. This is the whole Torah; all the rest is commentary. Go and learn it. *Hillel, Talmud, Shabbath 31a*

- ***Native American:*** We are as much alive as we keep the earth alive. *Chief Dan George*

Extend Ahimsa toward all of creation.

- Extend Ahimsa toward yourself too by developing a sense of non-violence in your actions, words, thoughts and intentions towards others and ourselves.

- We may practice non-violence in our actions, words, thoughts and intentions towards others. But we may punish ourselves when we sense failure.

- We must avoid the illusion of perfection, which brings violence towards oneself. Perfection is not possible; it is an illusion. Perfection is not necessary for love.

As we saw earlier in Forgiveness, Ahimsa extends toward all creation, not just others. It extends towards the self. Therefore, do not punish yourself over your perceived failures. Do not hold yourself to a perfect example. Perfection is not necessary for love. Love yourself for your flaws as well as your strengths.

Because we are all one.

The Brihadaranyaka Upanishad 4.12 says "As a lump of salt thrown in water dissolves and cannot be taken out again, though wherever we taste, the water is salty, even so, beloved, the separate self dissolves in the sea of pur consciousness, infinite and immortal."

We are all one and cannot be separated. Therefore, what you do to another you do to yourself. We are all one. Ahimsa extended toward one extends toward all including the self. As salt dissolves in water, it makes the water salty but cannot be separated again. We are like that salt. Or seen another way, you can take a drop of water out of the ocean, but that drop is still the ocean. You are connected to all there is. Therefore, whatever you do to another, you do to yourself.

Self Care – Practice Saucha to support Ahimsa.

The first of the Niyamas is Saucha or cleanliness, also called purity. Although, typically, the Niyamas are separate from the Yamas, if we are to extend Ahimsa to ourselves, then Saucha is one of the ways we do that.

- Saucha translates as purity. This is often reduced to cleanliness or a lack of excess. It's important to keep the outside of the body clean by washing frequently; to keep the inside of the body pure by eating and drinking moderately and choosing food and drink that is clean, healthy and fortifying; and to maintain order in our living and working spaces.

- But in its truest sense as a niyama, or observance, saucha refers to a pure situation engendered by our actions, a situation wherein unwanted things don't appear and the conditions for goodness and happiness do. This situation of purity created by our actions we can then notice and experience.

By living in a clean and uncluttered environment, keeping our body and clothes clean and eating clean food, we maintain health and vibrancy. This is good not only for us, but for those around us as in a state of health, we can serve. Poor hygiene, a cluttered environment and unhealthy food make us unable to serve others. Indeed, they lead us to be a burden. But don't be too judgmental about this condition. Again, perfection is not required. Use discernment to decide the optimum conditions for your health and environment.

Practice Saucha in thought, word and deed.

- If we intend purity in thought, word and deed, then we create the least amount of suffering for ourselves and for others.

- Examine the intention behind your words. THINK:

  - ♥ Is it true.
  - ♥ Is it helpful.
  - ♥ Is it necessary.
  - ♥ Is it kind.

Female Yoga master Judith Lassiter mentions that the idea of purity was off-putting to her because it sounds pretty judgmental. When interpreted rigidly, it can be tempting to place everything into one of two categories: pure or impure. I should eat this food, but not that. I can hang out with him, but not her. I'm allowed to think these kinds of thoughts, but not those. But are things ever so black and white? No. Don't be too judgmental about this condition.

Again, perfection is not required. Use discernment to decide the optimum conditions for your health and environment.

Learn and practice Feng Shui.

The Chinese practice of Feng Shui can help us to create a physical environment that conforms to the practice of Saucha. Feng Shui is an ancient Chinese practice that uses the energy of the five elements, fire, water, wood metal and air to balance the dynamics of an environment.

The Chinese practice of Feng Shui is integral to Saucha. Feng Shui asks us to create an environment that allows energy to flow. Feng shui seeks to promote prosperity, good health, and general well being by optimizing energy flow through a living environment

- ♥ Keep your house free of clutter.
- ♥ Clear a path to the front door
- ♥ Give guests a reason to pause and admire.
- ♥ Balance the five elements—fire, water, wood, metal and air.
- ♥ Remove negative symbolism.
- ♥ Maximize natural light.

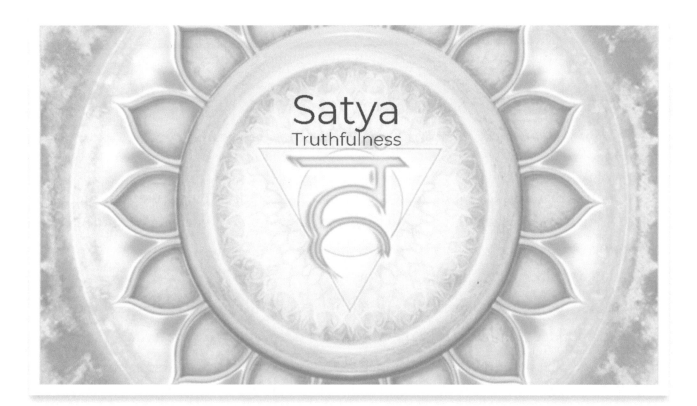

Chapter 4: Satya— Truthfulness.

You may think truth is easy to discern and practice. But is it?

Book two of Patanjali's Yoga Sutras Chapter 36

- ***To one established in truthfulness, actions and their results become subservient.***

Remember that Sanskrit words are often the source of words in Indo-European languages, including English. Sat, then, is the root for the English word *such* which is a word that alludes definition:

Dictionary.com says *such* means "of a kind."

American Heritage Dictionary adds "itself alone or within itself."

The Cambridge Dictionary calls the word *such* a determiner—whatever that means.

In Sanskrit the definition of Sat is much the same as *such*. Sat is of an entity, species or existence and variously implies that which is true, being, happening, real, existing, enduring, lasting, essential.

Thus, Sat is the *such*ness of a thing, its existence, its essence, its eternal being.

Is it not similar to "I am that am", the name of God, the infinite consciousness of the universe?

Thus, in observing Satya I can say of myself, "I am not a female human. I am not my long list of career accomplishments. I am not even the multiplicity of cells and microbes which make up the temple into which my existence projects. I am a projection of infinite consciousness focused into a field of time and space where I share the experiences of existence with other such projections." There's that word such again.

I, therefore, undefine myself from any illusion of materiality that separates me from the infinite. I am surrendered to the infinite, allowing it to bring me into the domain of pure potential from which I can choose, with my focused consciousness, I can choose my experience on a momentary basis using time as my creative medium.

- Swami Satchidnanda, who is the Yoga master who translated the edition of the Yoga Sutras that I am referencing. comments about truthfulness in terms of Law of Attraction. He says, "Nature loves an honest person. By telling the truth all the time, even abstaining from white lies, blessings will follow you. He mentions that this also means if being honest causes harm, then say nothing."

Patanjali says that actions and results follow truth. Swami Satchidananda, in his comments on Satya, says that blessings and abundance follow truth. He reminds us not even to tell white lies, but say nothing if we feel it necessary to tell a white lie.

- TKV Desikachar says, "Speak only pleasant truths so that Satya does not come at the expense of Ahimsa." Referring to the Mahabharata, he quotes, "Speak the Truth which is pleasant. Do not speak unpleasant truths. Do not lie, even if the lies are pleasing to the ear. That is the dharma." He also connects Satya with Law of Attraction saying when one is established in truth, those things he needs come to him.

Desikachar reminds us not to forget Ahimsa in our truthfulness. Desikachar echos Swami Satchidananda when he cautions us to say nothing if your truth will hurt, that, saying not to lie even if the lie sounds pleasant. He rfers us to Dharma. Dharma is the law that governs life. Dharma is truth, even if we do not like the truth. But we needn't express that truth in harmful words. So, is it helpful, is it necessary, is it kind. Sometimes truth is none of those.

- BKS Iyengar says truth is the highest rule of conduct and quotes Ghandi: "Truth is God and God is Truth. Truth cleanses the Yogi and burns the dross in him. In perfect truth, one becomes fit for union with the Infinite." He refers to abuse, obscenity, falsehoods, calumny, gossip and ridicule as poison.

In other words, you cannot meet that infinite field of all there is if you are living in falsehoods and lies, including obscenity, calumny, gossip and ridicule.

- American Yoga master Donna Fahri expresses the feminine perspective. She extends Satya to yourself, saying that it means leaving unhealthy relationships and coming out of your comfort zone. She says truth brings inner peace. She reminds us that Satya also means leaving unhealthy relationships.

We might think we know the truth, but in human culture, truth is a moving target.

We think we know truth but consider this:

- ♥ In the 16th and 17th centuries, Galileo Galilei's theory that the earth revolves around the sun was declared to be "foolish and absurd in philosophy, and formally heretical since it explicitly contradicts in many places the sense of Holy Scripture." He was imprisoned for going against the "truth" of the day.
- ♥ In the 18th century, medicine used blood letting as a cure.
- ♥ In the 20th century, cigarettes were considered healthy, as were many other substances now known to cause cancer.

Truth, facts, science, these change over time. So is there even one truth? And is that even truth, or just an agreement among authorities? Truth, then, seems dependent on the consensus of the current authorities or experts.

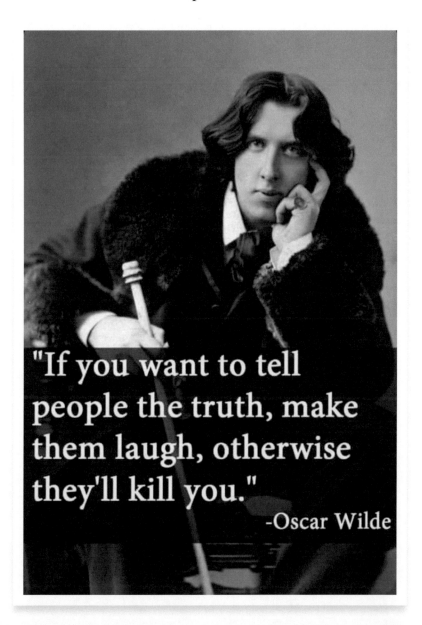

Indeed, we live in a ocean of untruths.

- ♥   We have to make people swear on a bible to tell the truth in court. "Do you swear to tell the truth, the whole truth, and nothing but the truth?"
- ♥   We carry identification to ensure we are who we say we are.

And politics is all about distrust and accusations.

- ♥   We have had a president who said about the truth "it depends on what your definition of is is."

We lie to our children from the day they are born.

My niece was adamant that her parents had lied to her when she was child. She was bitter and angry even until she became an adult. She told me her anger was because they lied to her about Santa Claus.

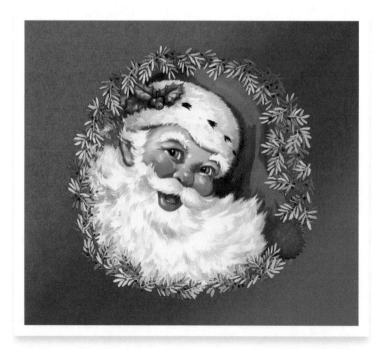

I recently asked her why she had carried that anger so long and still carries it; she is now 41 years old. She told me that she had thought of Santa Claus as someone real who loved her. One Christmas, when she was about 6, she was complaining that Santa loved her more than her Dad because he gave her better presents. Upon hearing that complaint, her mother said to her,

"Honey, your dad is Santa."

At that point, my niece told me that she felt as if someone who loved her and whom she loved had died. She felt a real loss and grieving with the revelation her mother had given her. From that, she questioned everything her parents told her that was not physically provable. So, how can we trust that which authorities tell us is true if even our parents start our lives based on lies?

We as children are bullied and gaslighted into obedience. Our parents, in their misguided attempt to make us conform utilize the worst form of lies to control us.

- ♥ They take away our toys.
- ♥ They intimidate, they tell us we are a disappointment,
- ♥ the bribe us with sweets and toys,
- ♥ they shame us,
- ♥ the judge us,
- ♥ and they gaslight us by telling us our feelings are "overreactions."

We are raised in an environment of lies to mold us into obedient socially acceptable creatures.

This leads to us not even knowing what the truth actually is. If we have been gaslighted or abused by authorities in our lives, we learn not to trust. Especially, we learn to lie if we are covering up for an abuser or gaslighter. Or maybe we feel shame about something that makes us feel "less than."

Often our shame comes from comparing ourselves to others and feeling envy to be like them or to have stuff like they do. We believe we have to aggrandize to get a job or gain status.

But you see, this is all from fear that you are not enough. And it starts in childhood. When we tell children that they are overreacting and do not validate their emotions, we begin to teach them to lie.

You are enough.

One thing that studying ancient knowledge teaches us is that we are loved as we are by the universe, regardless of our lacks, in fact because of our lacks. Each of us is unique and loved. The Bhagavad Gita is the love song of God and teaches us that we are loved. It is only doubt of our lovability that causes us fear and makes us lie.

It is difficult process to find your truth in our fear and lie based society.

Practice Svadyaya to support Satya

Svadyaya is the practice of –

- ♥ self-study,

- ♥ self-awareness,

- ♥ self-knowledge,

- ♥ self-reflection,

- ♥ self-examination.

In Sanskrit, *Sva* means "self" or "belonging to me", while *Adhyaya* means "inquiry," "examination," or "education." Education is the drawing out of the best that is within a person. Svadhyaya, therefore, is the education of the self.

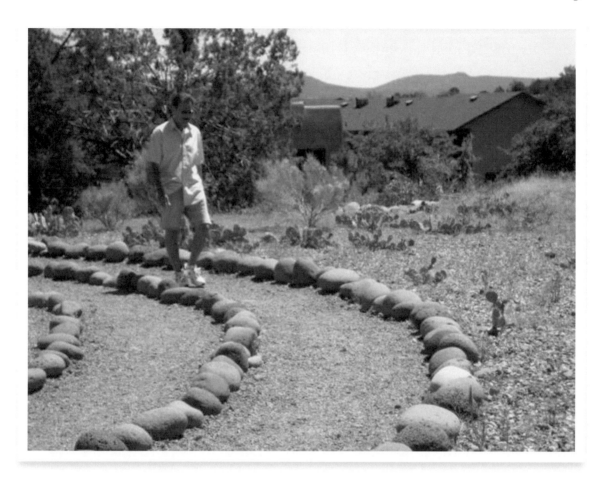

B.K.S. Iyengar says

The person practicing Svadhyaya reads his own book of life, at the same time that he writes and revises it. There is a change in his outlook on life. He starts to realize that there is divinity within himself, and that the energy which moves him is the same that moves the entire universe.

In Yoga, Svadyaya is self-examination. It is one of the Niyamas or spiritual practices that ushers us toward meditation by giving us contentment with who we are as a person. Svadyaya guides us to look at ourselves objectively.

Svadyaya takes effort. It takes a close, objective, look at ourselves that includes becoming aware of those aspects of yourself that you do not like. In modern terms, the aspects of yourself that you do not like are commonly called your **Shadow**.

The psychologist Carl Jung coined the term **Shadow** to refer to one of the main archetypes residing in the personal unconscious that have the most disturbing effects on the Ego.

Jung wrote:

> "The Shadow is a moral problem that challenges the whole Ego-personality, for no one can become conscious of the Shadow without considerable moral effort. To become conscious of it involves recognizing the dark aspects of the personality as present and real."

This is not an easy task. Jung goes on to add, "This act is an essential condition for any kind of self-knowledge and it therefore, as a rule, meets with considerable resistance."

The resistance comes from our emotional reaction to those dark aspects. To admit we have those traits makes us unlovable, and we all want love. Thus, when we see ourselves as mean, lazy, gluttonous, lecherous, greedy, aggrandizing, or envious, we fear that we are unlovable and therefore unloved and that is a difficult blow to our ego.

Yet, we see those traits in others quite easily in a mental process psychologists call "projection." In other words, in order to protect our ego from being unloved, we project those qualities that we fear most about ourselves onto others. We project our Shadow onto others. We see the characteristics of our Shadow in other people. Have you ever had to interact with someone who just drives you up the wall? Have you had to be around someone who was mean, condescending, and self-aggrandizing? How about someone who shuts you down before you have had a chance to speak? I know I have.

Recently, I had to attend meetings with a person who was so toxic to me that it took me a day to get over it. I was angry, hurt, unable to function. I felt sick and was unable to do my work or enjoy any leisure. I had to find a way to cope with my feelings, otherwise, this interaction would paralyze me. So I turned to Yoga to find the way. I turned to the Yamas and Niyamas. I had faith that practicing the Niyama Svadyaya would help me find my way.

Practicing Svadyaya made me look at my own Shadow relative to the person who had vexed me. When I judged that person to be toxic—mean, condescending and aggrandizing—I knew I must be projecting those traits and that they were attributes that I fear most about myself.

Was I, in fact, mean? Did I condescend to others? Was I aggrandizing and did I shut others down? I reached back into my memory to find times when I had done so. They weren't hard to find.

I am mean. I had been mean recently. I had said some extremely mean things about another person, in fact, about that person! I'm not physically mean. I don't kill or hurt anything. I'm one of those people who escorts spiders out of the house on a piece of paper. When it rains, I pick worms up off the sidewalk and place them on the dirt. But my thoughts can be dark and my words can cut deeply.

I have condescended to people. I condescended to my niece when she was a little girl. I aggrandize. Aggrandizing was a critique I received on a work review once. And I do shut others down, especially if I think they are less intelligent than I am.

I found, through Svadyaya, that I had all the qualities I had projected on the person who drove me up the wall. Indeed, that person is a reflection of me, of my Shadow. In that person, I confronted my own Shadow and I didn't like it—at all.

My practice of Svadyaya reminded me that I am still a work in progress. Indeed, B.K.S. Iyengar's idea of Svadyaya as "reading your own book-of-life at the same time as writing and revising it" fit with this experience exactly. It is time for me to do a bit of revision. It is time for me to recognize my Shadow, accept it, and recognize that when I judge someone else harshly, it is likely because I see something in that person that I don't like in myself.

How about you? Can you read, write and revise your book of life considering your Shadow? I hope this book helps you to do so.

Asteya
Non-Stealing

Chapter 5 Asteya— Non-stealing

Book two of Patanjali's Yoga Sutras, Chapter 37

♥ *To one established in non-stealing, all wealth comes.*

- *If we are completely free from stealing and greed, contented with what we have, and if we keep serene minds, all wealth comes to us.*

The principle behind Asteya is found throughout spiritual and religious practices. Many practices teach that the higher power (or your higher self) supplies what you need in any moment. If you are content in the "eternal now," the only moment that is, you will always have all you need.

This concept is echoed in the Judeo-Christian psalms and prayers. The 23rd psalm says "I shall not want." The Christian "Lord's Prayer" says "Give us this day our daily bread," asking the higher power to give us, in this moment what we need. These teachings can be seen as lessons in mindfulness and in being present in the moment. If you are mindful of each moment and present in that moment, you will be aware of what you have and what you need in that moment. When we are not secure in each moment, we look to the future with fear. We are afraid we will not have enough in each moment to survive, so we hoard our "stuff."

In the translation of the Yoga Sutras, Swami Satchidananda talks about non-stealing in terms of Law of Attraction. He says when you are content with what you have, with a serene mind, all wealth comes to you. He says do not hoard or lock your "stuff" away because then it wants to get out, but let it flow freely so it wants to stay with you. And share your stuff.

Asteya teaches us to take life each moment at a time. It teaches us that if we have more in this moment, to share with others. It teaches that if we have money or other things that can be put to use to help those in need, then we should share it with them. In that way, we become an agent of God who provides for the wants of others and the daily bread of others.

This includes the sharing of knowledge. That is why we become teachers.

- ♥ TKV Desikachar just says don't take what's not yours. Don't' take advantage of other people.
- ♥ BKS Iyengar talks about envy and craving including mismanagement, breach of trust, misappropriation, misuse. He also refers to the commandment, "Thou shalt not steal." Also, "Thou shalt not covet thy neighbor's goods."
- ♥ The Yoga masters go a bit beyond stealing and hoarding by mentioning envy and craving, mismanagement, and breach of trust, as stealing.
  - Stealing is the Deadly Sin "Greed or Avarice"
  - It is covetousness as in the hoarding of materials or objects,
  - It is theft or robbery.
  - It is especially manipulation by authority.

Why do we steal?

- **We steal out of fear that we don't have enough. We lock our wealth away to ensure it is there for us when we need it.**

- **Yet, locking up our money and things is a form of stealing. The money and things are not put to use to benefit others, but removed from use. This act steals usefulness from money and things that could serve others and encourages those who do not have as much to take what we have.**

How else do we steal besides stealing and hording of goods? What beyond things do we steal.

♥ **Gossip is stealing reputation.**

We steal non-material things from people by stealing their reputation through gossip.

♥ **Being late is stealing time**.

We steal time when we are late.

♥ **Not listening is stealing energy and time.**

We steal energy when we do not listen. How many times have you been in a conversation where you are formulating what you are going to say next while your companion is still talking. You are stealing their energy and time when you do that. If you are mindful and live in the moment, you will listen to your companion.

We also steal when we cheat.

And usually cheating is stealing from yourself. You cheat because you do not trust your own ability. You do not trust your connection to the higher self. Cheating happens at school when we copy or plagiarize because we fear failing. You may cheat at a game or sport because you doubt your own ability to win. You may cheat on your significant other, thus destroying a relationship.

This refers back to Satya. If you are truthful, you do not steal or cheat.

Santosa, practice Santosa to support Asteya

- ♥ Santosa in Sanskrit, derived from San meaning "completely", "altogether" or "entirely", and Tosa, "contentment", "satisfaction", "acceptance", "being comfortable".

- ♥ When we are content with what we have, we feel secure and have no need to take what is not ours.

- ♥ Our contentment allows our self esteem to grow. We gain faith in our own ability to create what we want.

Santosa is a Niyama that supports Asteya. Santosa means to be content in the moment. By being content, we accept what we have and feel secure in the moment. Contentment leads to self esteem, so that we do not feel the need to covet or be greedy. We do not need to cheat, and we can be attentive to others so as not to steal their time or energy. Spirit is also connected to "now." It will ride into your imagination through whatever gives you pleasure in this moment so pay attention to what brings you pleasure now, not at another time, but right now. Whatever you are drawn to most in this moment is where spirit is. To borrow from Jeff Foxworthy: If you really want to buy that ice cream cone, you may want to pay attention to everything connected to that act. If you are drawn to a day at the beach, you might want to pay attention. If that puppy at the pet store has "your name written on it," you may be hearing from spirit. Likewise, if you hear a popular song in your head, pay attention to the lyrics. Pay attention to everything that's happening in your mind-space and physical space in the now, for that space is the stage on which spirit is acting to get your attention.

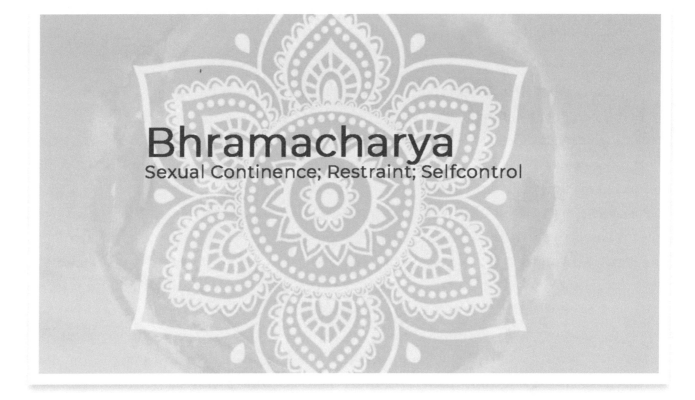

Chapter 6 Bhramacharya— Continence

Book two of Patanjali's Yoga Sutras Chapter 38

♥ *To one established in (sexual) continence, vigor is gained.*

The translator of the Yoga Sutras that I am referencing, Swami Satchidananda, talks about sexual continence in terms of retaining energy. He emphasizes celibacy, thus reserving sex only for marriage and then only to make babies.

Bramacharya is about sexual continence, or restraint, something that has been abandon in our modern culture. Whether you agree with sexual restraint or not, the idea is that sex is a spiritual, energetic exchange not to be taken lightly. Sex is an exchange of energy that binds you, at the quantum level, to your sex partner. Care should be taken about whom you exchange energy with.

The yoga masters say this about Bhramacharya:

- *TKV Desikachar goes further to say that one should keep intimacy for relationships to foster our highest truth and respect the family.*
- *BKS Iyengar talks about the Bhramachari as "one who is engrossed in study of divinity, thus has little time or interest in pleasures of the flesh."*

The Yoga masters are concerned with Brhamacharya as it respects family life. Indeed, Brhamacharya says that sex is only acceptable within marriage to support family life, which is also the emphasis of the feminine perspective. Yoga tradition divides life into four cycles, where the third is raising a family. In the other cycles, yoga says one should not participate in sexual activity.

In the Western Judeo-Christian culture, we see Bhramacharya expressed as the the deadly sin of lust.

Lust is usually thought of as intense or unbridled sexual desire, which leads to fornication, adultery, rape, bestiality, and other sinful sexual acts.

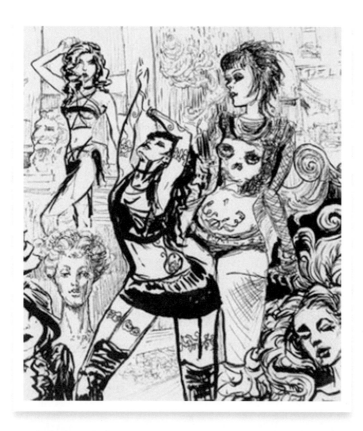

The thing that is so attractive about sexual activity, besides the thrill of orgasm, is that the sex act releases Oxytocin, a neurotransmitter that makes you think you are in love. But the reality is that you are only responding to a chemical reaction in your brain. Have you ever thought you were in love with someone who satisfied you sexually only to find out the other person didn't love you? I probably don't have to tell you how bac that feels. You feel hurt, even violated and sometimes dirty. Or maybe you are the object of another's love and you can't return it. So you are the one who is hurtful, the violator, the dirty one.

Sexual predation, seeking out and using someone for immediate gratification, is not unusual, but it is hurtful on many different levels. This is especially true when the predator is more powerful than the prey. Our culture is no longer tolerant of such activity among powerful people. Yet, the predators defend themselves and blame their prey.

And pedophilia goes on in the darkest corners of our culture, the dirtiest secret that no one wants to talk about, leaving the most innocent injured beyond repair, or dead.

Sex has consequences that for which Bhramacharya asks us to take responsibility.

The consequences can be much greater than just cultural violations and hurt feelings, as I am sure you already know. There is disease, which can be very serious. In today's world, we have cures for sexually transmitted diseases, but that wasn't always true. Up until the early 20th century, syphilis was easily transmitted and deadly. We all know the consequences of the AIDS epidemic in the late 20th century. Now, we have ways to combat and even cure these diseases, but still doesn't mean we should take them for granted.

And of course there is pregnancy. In today's world, women have reproductive rights which means they have access to effective birth control and abortion, even late term abortion. Yet, no woman in her right mind ever obtained an abortion without emotional pain, not to mention bodily trauma, not matter what the current media tells you.

Bhramacharya asks us not to abort our children. Yet, unwanted children also suffer. They are most likely to be abused, neglected and trafficked.

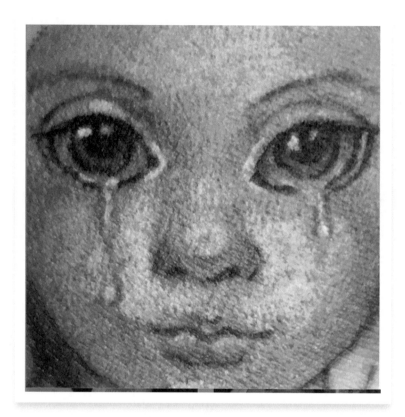

Speaking about Bhramacharya is a challenge in our culture. Indeed, when one of my teachers who was presenting an online workshop on the Yamas and Niyamas came to Bhramacharya, he said, "sex has consequences and I will leave it at that." Privately, I called him out on that cop-out and he explained to me how hard it was for him, a man, to be in a Yoga class with a group of modern women explaining to them why they should refrain from casual sex, not use birth control or abortion. I felt for him, but still thought it to be a major cop-out. Here he was teaching Yoga, "yoking with the infinite" without explaining that one cannot reach the peace of mind necessary to yoke with the infinite when one is carrying the type of guilt, shame and fear associated with the consequences of a sexual relationship gone bad.

Guilt, shame, and fear can be avoided simply by being discerning in one's sexual encounters.

Again, this boils down to Ahimsa and thinking about what you are doing in terms of non-violence. Consider if the sexual relationship you have one that is seated firmly in loving kindness.

What about lusting after other things such as money, drugs or power?

Should we not apply Bhramacharya to those lusts as well? Indeed, Bhramachary also applies to unbridled desire in general. In Judeo-Chistian culture the seven deadly sins say that the impurity of lust transforms one into "a slave of the devil".

- ♥ **Drugs and alcohol**
- ♥ **Compulsive repetitive behaviors**
- ♥ **Rage**
- ♥ **Obsessions**
- ♥ **Gambling**

We may refer to these as addictions that have serioius negatve impact on your life and the lives of those around you.

Practice Tapas to help with Bhramacharya.

There is a Niyama that can help with the self-control needed to practice Bhramacharya. That Niyama is Tapas.

- ♥ Tapas translates as austerity or discipline.
- ♥ The word Tapas is derived from the root Sanskrit verb 'tap' which means 'to burn' and evokes a sense of 'fiery discipline' or 'passion'.

♥ Tapas can mean cultivating a sense of self-discipline, passion and courage in order to burn away 'impurities' physically, mentally and emotionally, and paving the way to our true greatness.

♥ Tapas is an aspect of the inner wisdom that encourages us to use restraint over behaviors that are self destructive.

♥ Tapas encourages us instead to engage in a practice such as Yoga on a regular basis.

Tapas is the Niyama that helps us control our lust and cravings. It literally refers to the burning off of those desires. It means self-discipline and even asks us to redirect our lust toward activity that supports us and uplifts us. Sigmund Freud, the father of psycho analysis, asks us to redirect sexual energy into creativity. Practicing Tapas helps us by giving us the discipline to do so.

By practicing the discipline of Asana and Pranayama we dispel the energy that may have been misdirected into lustful activity.

Tapas asks us to engage in a regular exercise routine or Yoga practice that includes Asana and Pranayama, breath control. By burning physical energy, we release endorphins, which are neuro-transmitters that make us feel calm and composed. Asana helps us to align our energy centers, chakra, and come closer to our higher self. This quells any obsessive compulsion we may have toward drug use, alcoholism, gambling, rage or predatory sex. We then have a calmer mind as we have no guilt or shame associated with such lustful activities.

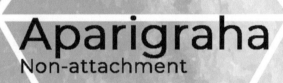

Aparigraha
Non-attachment

Chapter 7 Aparigraha—Non-attachment; letting go of that which no longer serves us

- Book two of Patanjali's Yoga Sutras Chapter 39

When non-greed is confirmed, a thorough illumination
of the how and why of one's birth comes.

Swami Satchidnanda talks about non-greed in terms of not accepting gifts as they oblige you to the giver. He clearly is talking about bribes here, not gifts as by accepting a gift, you allow the giver to express loving kindness. By rejecting a gift, you may cause harm and emotional pain to the giver. Swami Satchidnanda talks about being free of desires and obligations. Accept gifts with good grace in a spirit of reciprocity, not obligation.

Aparigraha relates closely to Asteya in that it requires one to be content with what one has. It requires that we let go of that which does not serve.

- TKV Desikachar also refers to not accepting gifts. He says we should only accept what we have earned. Again, he is referring to bribes, not something freely given in loving kindness.

- BKS Iyengar relates Aparigraha to Asteya. He says that when one hoards, it shows a lack of faith that God will provide. He relates it to the waxing and waning of the moon: that even when it is waning, it does not stray from its course.

- The feminine perspective asks us not be grasping and possessiveness. By grasping for status symbols such as designer bags, shoes, jewelry, we are acting out of insecurity. If

Buddhism, which is an offshoot of Yoga, teaches non-attachment. Attachment causes suffering.

- ♥ **When we are attached to our stuff, we live in fear of loss.**
- ♥ **When we are attached to our significant other, we become jealous.**
- ♥ **When we are attached to stuff people and outcomes, we block energy and prevent our ability to manifest that which will serve us better.**
- ♥ **Indeed, when we attach to outcomes, we are never satisfied.**

Some years ago, I attended a matinée at an art theatre in uptown Washington, DC. As I approached the entrance, under the marquee, seated leaning against the show window, was a woman who appeared to be homeless. She was dirty, a bit disheveled and surrounded by some bags, which ostensibly contained her worldly possessions.

"Spare change?," she said to me as I passed.

"I'm sorry, I have no change, but look," I said pointing out a nickel, a dime and two pennies that were sitting on the sidewalk just in front of her. "There's some money right there. Take that!"

Upon that suggestion, she made a devilish face and, pushing the money aside, growled, "I can't do anything with that!"

I was quite taken aback. After all, she had asked for spare change and certainly seventeen cents qualified as spare change. So, picking the money up, I said, "well, I can." And I put the coins in my pocket. At that time in my life, my money was a bit tight and I wasn't going to pass up free money. As luck would have it, that seventeen cents gave me just enough to buy popcorn.

By shoving the money away, the homeless woman was expressing discontent with the outcome she expected. She was not satisfied with what was right in front of her. It is attachment to outcome that causes the most suffering.

Santosa—Practice Santosa to support Aparigraha.

The Niyama Santosa tells us to be content with what we have in the moment.

In Chapter 5, we talked about Santosa as it supports Asteya, non-stealing. Recall that in Sanskrit, the word Santosa is derived from San meaning "completely", "altogether" or "entirely", and Tosa, "contentment", "satisfaction", "acceptance", "being comfortable".

- ♥ **By living in each present moment, we generate the next moment of contentment as we push through the leading edge of time.**

- ♥ **Christianity asks the universe to give us each "day" our bread. It tells us to not want as the universe will take care of each want as it arises.**

ISVARA PRANIDANA
Surrender to Infinite Source

Chapter 8 Isvara Pranidana— Surrender to infinite source

"In a real sense faith is total surrender to God."
Martin Luther King, Jr

Patanjali mentions Isvara Pranidana, the final Niyama, in the first book and the second book of the *Yoga Sutras*. It is that important.

♥ Book one Chapter 23—***Samadhi is attained by devotion with total dedication to Isvara*** (Infinite Source)

♥ Book one Chapter 24—***Isvara is the supreme Purusha (non-material substance) unaffected by afflictions, actions, fruits of actions or by any inner impressions of desires.***

♥ Book two Chapter 45—By total surrender to infinite source, samadhi is attained.

Ishvara Pranidhana is an ultimate in the practice of Yoga. It initiates a sacred shift of perspective that helps us to remember, align with, and receive the grace of becoming one with our higher self, with pure source energy. It brings us into Samadhi.

Ishvara Pranidhana is surrender to that higher source. To many modern Westerners the idea of surrender as a virtue may seem strange. Many of us have only experienced surrendering to a higher source as a **last resort**, when we've confronted seemingly insurmountable problems or in some other way hit the edge of our individual will and abilities.

In the *Yoga Sutras*, Patanjali transforms "surrender" from this sort of last-resort, emergency response into an essential ongoing practice. Patanjali repeatedly highlights Ishvara Pranidhana as the ultimate of the five Niyamas,

When we arrive at the practice of Isvara Pranidana, we yoke to infinite source through our surrender. Our ego recedes and is eclipsed by our higher self. We are thus able to communicate with the infinite. Infinite source hears us and always answers, "yes." We may call the answer we hear the voice of "Spirit."

Spirit communicates with us in any way it can to get our attention. Sometimes Spirit uses the words of a popular song. Sometimes it uses images. Sometimes it sends an emissary in the form of a spiritual guide. Sometimes it sends an emissary in the form of another person, or an animal, or a flower, or a picture. Sometimes it sends you on a trip you had no intention of taking, just perhaps to the store, where you find exactly what you need in the moment.

The point is, when our minds are free of clutter caused by fear-based emotions, we are able to hear infinite source speak through Spirit in many ways and in many forms. It doesn't necessarily give us dictation as it did for Neal Donald Walsh in his book series *Talking to God*. In fact, Spirit probably talks to Walsh in many different ways while Walsh waits and waits for his message to come through in writing.

The first time I was aware of Spirit actually talking to me, it spoke in French. It said. "Lève tes yeux. Tes yeux sont dans le caniveau." I knew a bit of French, but did not know the word, caniveau, so I looked it up. It means gutter. I knew then that the voice I heard was not my own ego's voice. I knew the message was coming from elsewhere. I had been sitting in meditation, seeking a message, but didn't expect it to come in words, much less in French. I expected something more subtle, a feeling or perhaps a dream or vision.

When you clear the way by eliminating the mind clutter, and you suspend disbelief and judgment by surrendering through the niyama of Isvara Pranadan, you are able to experience yoking with infinite source. You are able to experiend Yoga.

If you want to hear spirit talk, you have to listen very closely and pay close attention to any sign given to you. Everything counts, especially urges.

This lesson was brought home to me by "the million-dollar peanut butter and jelly sandwich." It didn't cost a million dollars, but it brought me a million dollars. Let me explain.

It happened while I resided in Paris. I had been living there for a year studying International Business Law at the American University of Paris. My tiny studio apartment was located in a beautiful area about a block from the Eiffel Tower. Every morning I jogged in the Champs de Mars, a grassy field that extends from the tower three blocks to the Avenue de la Motte Picquet across from the Ecole Militaire.

Paris is a beautiful city, as beautiful as its reputation. I was enchanted with Paris and didn't want to leave. I had lived there before, spoke French well and could navigate Paris easily by Metro and bus. In February, my course at the University ended and I faced the prospect of leaving the city I loved and returning "home" to the U.S. with nothing there—no job and no place to live. In fact, I would have to move back into my parents' home! Yikes! The idea made me very sad.

I had a student visa that would allow me to stay an additional six months if I could find a job. So set out to find a job I did. I scoured the job postings in the local newspaper and at the student center. I sent out dozens of hand-written letters (the French analyze your handwriting as part of the application), in French! I networked. I went to the student employment center and got a two-week gig working eight solid hours a day decorating baby shoes for a local artisan. But that gig wasn't good enough to satisfy the requirements of my visa, so I kept on searching.

Then one gloomy Sunday at the end of February, I decided to take the day off and just do what I wanted to do. I found that I had a craving for a peanut butter and jelly sandwich. Now, in France at the time, the early 1990s, there was no peanut butter or grape jelly in French stores. The bread available was baguettes and grand pains in long crusty loaves, or specialty bread in wheels. There was no soft, pasty, white Wonder Bread. That is, there was no peanut butter, no jelly and no American style white bread anywhere except a store called The Real McCoy located on the American University campus.

The Real McCoy specialized in catering to home-sick American students on study-abroad semesters at the University. It sold American food products such as Heinz ketchup and baked beans, Campbell's soup, Jello, peanut butter—both Skippy and Peter Pan–and Welch's grape jelly at premium prices. The clerks who worked there would make you a peanut butter and jelly sandwich on white bread for 45 francs. (It was before the Euro became the currency.) At one Franc equal to 20 cents, that price was $9.00—pretty high for a peanut butter and jelly sandwich.

No matter the cost, I had to have one. My job search had been exhausting and I needed something to make me feel like "home." My imagined sense of gooey, grapey glop oozing between my teeth and sticking to the roof of my mouth brought me a secure feeling, the ease of childhood, a feeling of being cared for, loved.

My money supply was meager. I didn't have 45 Francs in my purse, so I searched between the sofa cushions for embedded coins and emptied every pocket of every coat and jacket. After searching every nook and cranny in my tiny apartment, I finally came up with the 45 Francs to buy my coveted sandwich and whisked off to the Real McCoy just a few blocks away.

Upon arrival, I ordered my peanut butter and jelly sandwich, "Peter Pan please, and Welch's grape jelly on Wonder bread," and forked over a handful of coins to pay. It was served to me on a napkin with a cup of water. I sat down at a counter beneath a bulletin board to savor the first bite. Sinking my teeth into the goo, I sighed as the sweet, salty gelatinous paste filled my mouth. In joyful satisfaction, I let my eyes wander to the bulletin board where I saw a card that said, "Help Wanted. English speaking computer operator. American papers OK." And a phone number.

Needless to say, the next day, I phoned the number, went for an interview and was hired. The job turned out to involve market research, which was something I had studied as a Psychology major. That job led to a subsequent series of high-level market research jobs paying, on average, $50,000 a year over the next twenty years, which totals one million dollars.

Had I not surrendered that day to do what I was urged to do, had I not acted on my urge, had I hesitated at the price of my desire, I would not have found that job and my life would have been different. Would it have been better? Would I have found another equal or better job? Who knows? But what I do know is this: Spirit, your higher self, that part of you that connects to the infinite, knows the way to your next best opportunity and will show it to you if you pay attention. Spirit will seek the path of least resistance to convey the message to you and that path is likely something which pleases you in the moment. If you turn your attention to that which will make you happy, act on the urge to be happy now, then you will find the next step to the next happiness and the next happiness over and over again.

Abraham Hicks tells you to "prepave" the road to your success by turning your attention to positive thoughts. By following the principles of the Yamas and practicing the Niyamas, we disengage from negativity and turn our attention to the positive. You act in loving kindness; you tell the truth, you don't steal things, time or reputation; you release that which doesn't serve you; you use discretion in your sexual activity. You stay clean in thought word and deed; you examine your life as you go along; you maintain a regular yoga practice; you are content in the moment. When you live with those practices, your mind is clear of guilt, shame, victimhood, revenge and all the other negative clutter that chatters. You are able to surrender to infinite source through your higher self and experience the syntropic emergence of that which you most desire in your life.

It will feel like you can dive into a swimming pool, reach out and pull the other side to you.

I hope this book serves you well. May you be happy and healthy.

The sacred light in me recognizes and honors the sacred light in you.

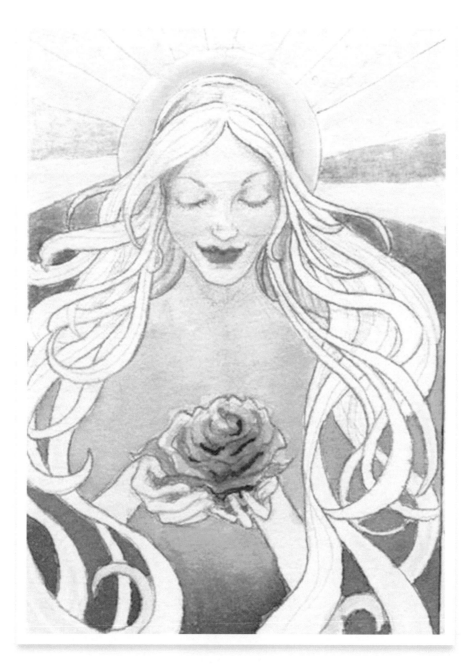

Namaste.

Sources and Resources

- The Heart of Yoga: Developing a Personal Practice by T. K. V. Desikachar
- Yoga Mind, Body & Spirit: A Return to Wholeness by Donna Farhi
- Light on Yoga: The Bible of Modern Yoga by B. K. S. Iyengar and Yehudi Menuhin
- The Upanishads, 2nd Edition Book 2 of 3: Easwaran's Classics of Indian Spirituality by Eknath Easwaran
- The Yoga Sutras of Patanjali by Sri Swami Satchidananda
- Bhagavad Gita: The Beloved Lord's Secret Love Song by Graham M. Schweig
- The Portable Jung (Portable Library) by C. G. Jung, Joseph Campbell, et al.

Special Thanks to

Nancy Ash and NewEarth University for motivating me to take on this project.

Risa Stevens for giving me use of her artwork.

Natasha Hennessey for teaching me Yoga.

Hari Kirtana Das for teaching Yoga philosophy.

Rodney and Colleen Yee for expanding my Yoga practice

Sacha Stone for inspiring me.

My dogs, Rowdy (at the rainbow bridge) and Toby

Printed in the United States
by Baker & Taylor Publisher Services